A REPORT OF THE CSIS
GLOBAL HEALTH POLICY CENTER

Global Health Policy in the Second Obama Term

Editor & Author
J. Stephen Morrison

Authors
Katherine E. Bliss
David Bowen
Nellie Bristol
Julie Fischer
Janet Fleischman
Amanda Glassman
Rebecca Katz
Hannah Kaye
Alisha Kramer
Phillip Nieburg
Sharon Stash
Todd Summers
Judyth Twigg

Editorial Coordinator
Matt Fisher

February 2013

50 YEARS | CHARTING OUR FUTURE

CSIS | CENTER FOR STRATEGIC & INTERNATIONAL STUDIES

About CSIS—50th Anniversary Year

For 50 years, the Center for Strategic and International Studies (CSIS) has developed solutions to the world's greatest policy challenges. As we celebrate this milestone, CSIS scholars are developing strategic insights and bipartisan policy solutions to help decisionmakers chart a course toward a better world.

CSIS is a nonprofit organization headquartered in Washington, D.C. The Center's 220 full-time staff and large network of affiliated scholars conduct research and analysis and develop policy initiatives that look into the future and anticipate change.

Founded at the height of the Cold War by David M. Abshire and Admiral Arleigh Burke, CSIS was dedicated to finding ways to sustain American prominence and prosperity as a force for good in the world. Since 1962, CSIS has become one of the world's preeminent international institutions focused on defense and security; regional stability; and transnational challenges ranging from energy and climate to global health and economic integration.

Former U.S. senator Sam Nunn has chaired the CSIS Board of Trustees since 1999. Former deputy secretary of defense John J. Hamre became the Center's president and chief executive officer in April 2000.

CSIS does not take specific policy positions; accordingly, all views expressed herein should be understood to be solely those of the author(s).

Cover photo: Getty Image by Mandel Ngan.

Center for Strategic and International Studies
1800 K Street, NW, Washington, DC 20006
Tel: (202) 887-0200
Fax: (202) 775-3199
Web: www.csis.org

2010[11] (see Figure 1). The WHO estimates that, without these investments, if the malaria incidence and mortality rates estimated for 2000 had remained unchanged over the decade, 274 million more cases and 1.1 million more deaths would have occurred between 2001 and 2010.[12]

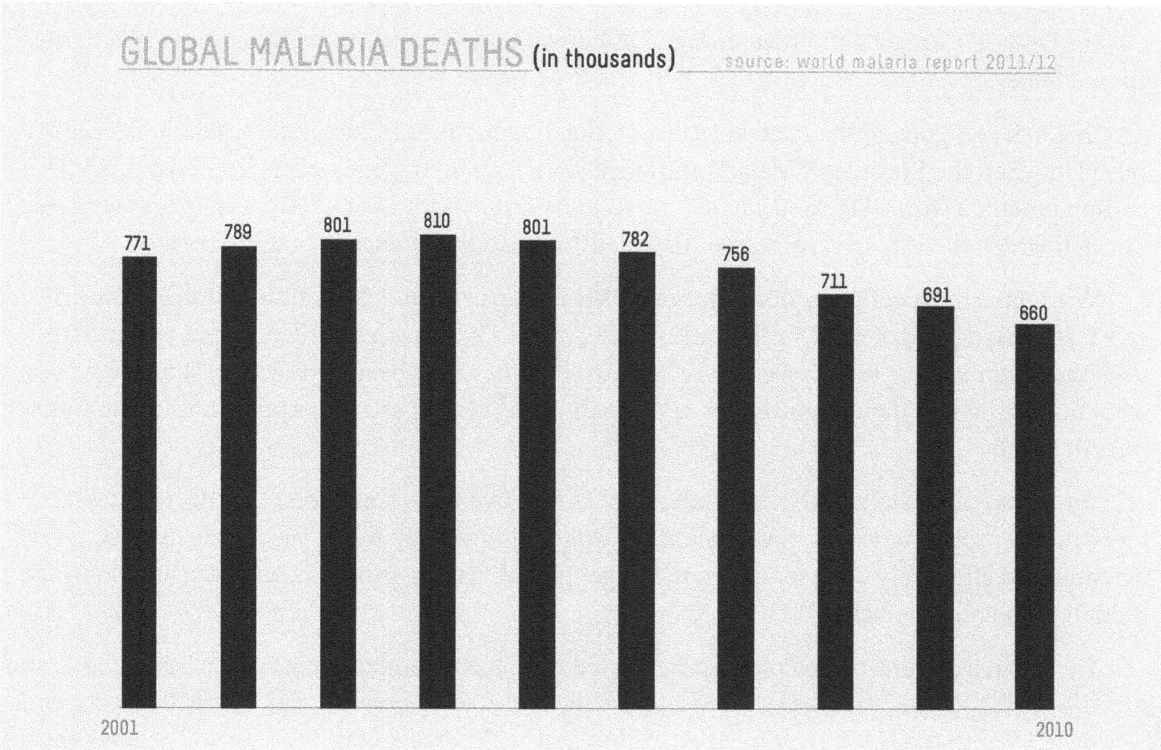

Today, 36 of the 99 remaining endemic countries are moving from controlled low-endemic malaria to elimination, though only four of these countries are in Africa.[13] Investing in malaria is bringing benefits far beyond health improvements. A 2011 study found that companies achieved a 28 percent return[14] when investing in malaria prevention programs for their employees, with a 94 percent reduction in malaria-related work absence.[15] An increasing range of companies, particularly in the oil and gas production, mining, and consumer goods sectors, are recognizing the need to invest in malaria control, not only as a humanitarian priority but as a business decision, and are making significant contributions to the fight.

Yet, these gains are still fragile. Status quo program implementation, lack of research and development, emerging drug and insecticide resistance, and reduced resources could all contribute to a dramatic reversal in the progress that has been achieved so far, with devastating consequences. A renewed commitment to malaria could support even more progress toward elimination and, ultimately, eradication. The growing list of countries advancing through pre-elimination and elimination stages demonstrates that this achievement is possible, despite the challenges.

---

11. World Health Organization, *World Malaria Report 2011.*

12. World Health Organization, *World Malaria Report 2012*, ix.

13. Global Health Group and Malaria Atlas Project, *Atlas of Malaria-Eliminating Countries, 2011* (San Francisco, CA: Global Health Group, October 2011), 5, http://www.malariaeliminationgroup.org/sites/default/files/atlas/global/Global-Atlas-2011.pdf; and Malaria Elimination Group, "Elimination Resources," http://www.malariaeliminationgroup.org/resources.

14. Roll Back Malaria Partnership, *Business Investing in Malaria Control: Economic Returns and a Healthy Workforce for Africa*, 9.

15. Ibid.

Policy Developments under the First Obama Administration

The United States has long viewed malaria control as in the national interest. Indeed, the Centers for Disease Control and Prevention (CDC) was originally established to fight malaria in the United States.[16]

In 2005, recognizing the strategic value of global reductions in malaria, President George W. Bush launched the President's Malaria Initiative (PMI), an interagency effort housed at USAID, co-implemented with CDC, and carried out in partnership with DOD, NIH, and other agencies, through which the U.S. government substantially increased its focus on malaria control.

With bipartisan congressional support, PMI has grown from $30 million and 15 countries in FY 2006 to a peak of $650 million in FY 2012[17] and 19 countries.[18] The Obama administration has set ambitious targets for future success. PMI has now been directed to "achieve Africa-wide impact by halving the burden of malaria in 70 percent of at-risk populations in sub-Saharan Africa."[19]

An independent, external evaluation of PMI's first five years concluded that PMI "quickly reoriented a problematic U.S. government malaria program, took it to a large scale quickly, efficiently, and effectively complemented the larger global malaria program, and contributed to the reduction in child mortality."[20]

The Obama administration has also supported the Global Fund to Fight AIDS, Tuberculosis and Malaria (GFATM). In 2012, the GFATM funded an estimated 40 percent of global malaria programs worldwide,[21] with the U.S. government providing nearly 25 percent of its funding and actively engaging in programmatic and governance reforms. Funding levels for the GFATM have risen since FY 2007, reaching $1.3 billion in FY 2012—a significant increase in a climate of fiscal austerity.

All these initiatives are part of the overarching Global Health Initiative, begun by the Obama administration in 2009 as an effort to coordinate sometimes-disparate global health programs to maximize their impact around a theme of improving maternal and child health. Although the administrative structure of the Global Health Initiative has changed since its inception, it remains a conceptual framework for the administration's global health efforts.

Ongoing Challenges

The successes in combating malaria these past 10 years have resulted in a profoundly changed landscape—one that holds great promise, but also peril. Just as the results of successful antimalarial efforts are quickly apparent, so are the costs of backsliding. Successful efforts to control malaria

---

16. Centers for Disease Control and Prevention, "CDC's Origins and Malaria," February 8, 2010, http://www.cdc.gov/malaria/about/history/history_cdc.html.

17. U.S. Congress, *Conference Report 112-331* to accompany H.R. 2055 (P.L. 112-74), December 2011, 1330.

18. President's Malaria Initiative, "The President's Malaria Initiative: Sixth Annual Report to Congress: Executive Summary," 3.

19. Ibid., 3.

20. Ibid., 4.

21. World Health Organization, *World Malaria Report 2012*, 15.

Figure 1. Actual and Pledged U.S. Contributions 2000–2014, as of September 2012[31]

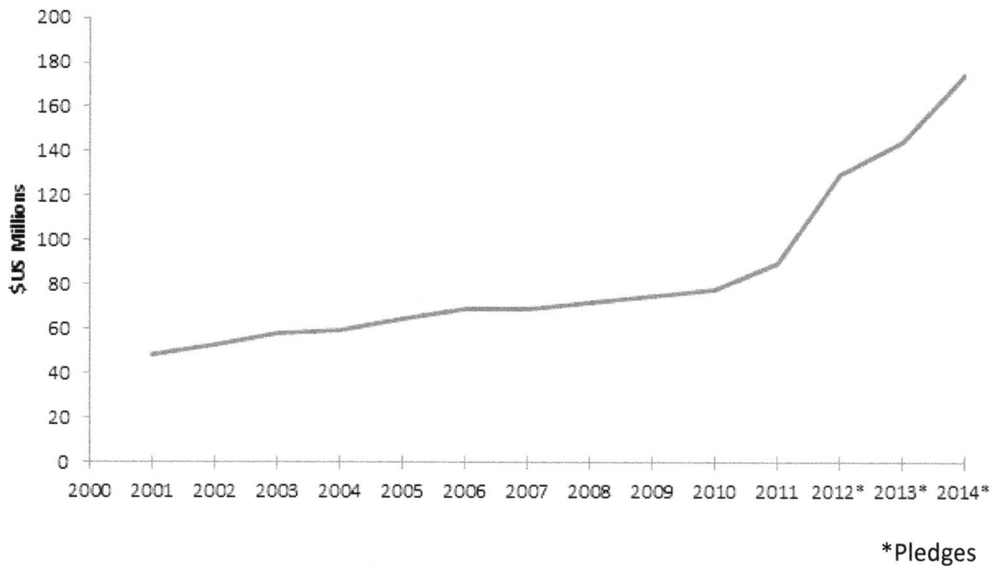

The United States represents Canada, Australia, Japan, and Korea on the GAVI Alliance board. The board is responsible for strategic direction and policymaking, oversees the operation of the Alliance, and monitors program implementation. During the second Obama administration, the board will oversee an important external evaluation of the Alliance's activities. It will also weigh measures to improve the quality of data, strengthen the incentives of partner governments to use vaccines more effectively, and better assess whether to adopt new cost-effective vaccines.

Policy Developments under the First Obama Administration

In recent years, following a difficult period of leadership change and funding uncertainty, GAVI has undergone a promising renewal.[32] During the GAVI Alliance's first pledging conference in June 2011, the United States pledged $450 million over three years (fiscal years 2012–2014) subject to congressional approval.[33] This represented a substantial increase over the previous year U.S. $90 million annual contribution. Overall, the replenishment was quite successful, with $4.3 billion pledged over five years. Meanwhile, a strong new chief executive officer, U.S. citizen Seth Berkley, and a new board chair, Norway's Dagfinn Høybråten, have generated a renewed sense of purpose and commitment among Alliance members.

31. GAVI Alliance, "Annual donor contributions to GAVI 2000–2031 as of 5 September 2012."

32. Lisa Carty, Amanda Glassman, Stephen Morrison, and Margaret Reeves, "GAVI'S Future: Steps to Build Strategic Leadership, Financial Sustainability, and Better Partnerships" (Washington, D.C.: CSIS, June 2011), http://csis.org/files/publication/110609_Carty_GAVI_0.pdf.

33. GAVI Alliance, "Donors commit vaccine funding to achieve historic milestone," June 13, 2011, http://www.gavialliance.org/library/news/press-releases/2011/donors-commit-vaccine-funding-to-achieve-historic-milestone-in-global-health/.

Due to U.S. Department of the Treasury and congressional objections,[34] the United States has not provided funding support to the GAVI Alliance's longer-term funding sources, the International Finance Facility for Immunization (IFFIm) and the Pneumococcal Vaccine Advanced Market Commitment (AMC).[35] These multiyear funding sources enable the Alliance to make longer-term commitments to countries and to vaccine manufacturers that can lead to reduced vaccine prices and quicker scale-up in country.

On the programmatic side, pneumococcal and rotavirus vaccines have been introduced in many GAVI-eligible countries, and although progress to date is slower than expected,[36] the pace is expected to increase and GAVI estimates that the introduction of the vaccine against pneumococcal disease in eligible countries could prevent approximately 500,000 premature deaths by 2015 and up to 1.5 million premature deaths by 2020, while the vaccine against rotavirus would prevent 2.4 million child deaths by 2030.[37]

The vaccine portfolio has recently been expanded to include vaccines against the human papilloma virus (HPV) and measles/rubella. The board has also agreed to future investments in vaccines against Japanese encephalitis and typhoid, when appropriate vaccines become available and have been reviewed by the World Health Organization (WHO). GAVI is also considering investments in additional vaccines, including inactivated poliovirus vaccine. An expert group supported by the GAVI secretariat—tasked with developing the next vaccine investment strategy[38]—will consider these proposed investments.

The 2002–2010 GAVI-initiated partnership with China to combat vaccine-preventable hepatitis B[39] was a notable achievement, increasing HepB3 coverage to more than 85 percent and timely birth dose vaccination coverage to more than 75 percent. In recent years, GAVI has expanded its efforts in Afghanistan, the Democratic Republic of Congo, and Somalia. The Democratic People's Republic of Korea has just launched the introduction of the five-antigens-in-one pentavalent vaccine, as has Myanmar. The pentavalent vaccine is a single vaccine that protects against diphtheria, pertussis, tetanus, hepatitis B, and Haemophilus influenzae type B, the bacterial microorganism that causes several serious childhood illnesses like meningitis and pneumonia.

GAVI has commissioned external evaluations to be conducted in five countries over 2013–2016, with the aim of generating real-time quantitative analysis of the relevance, effectiveness, impact, efficiency, and sustainability of GAVI support.

---

34. Benjamin Leo, *Can Donors Be Flexible within Restrictive Budget Systems? Options for Innovative-Financing Mechanisms*, Working Paper 226 (Washington, D.C.: Center for Global Development, October 2010), http://www.cgdev.org/files/1424497_file_Leo_Budget_Systems_Paper_FINAL.pdf.

35. IFFIm, *The International Finance Facility for Immunisation: Annual Report of the Trustees; Annual Financial Statements: Year Ended 31 December 2010*, http://www.iffim.org/finance/trustees-reports-and-financial-statements/; and GAVI Alliance, *Progress Report 2011* (Geneva: GAVI Alliance, 2011), http://www.gavialliance.org/results/gavi-progress-reports/.

36. Rotavirus vaccines have been rolled out in 9 countries since 2011, and to date, 18 countries have begun the introduction of pneumococcal vaccines. GAVI Alliance, "Vaccine goal indicators," http://www.gavialliance.org/results/goal-level-indicators/vaccine-goal-indicators/.

37. GAVI Alliance, "Factsheet: Advance Market Commitment," 2012; GAVI Alliance, "Factsheet: Rotavirus disease," 2012.

38. The board will consider this strategy at the end of 2013.

39. GAVI Alliance, "China's dramatic fall in hepatitis B infections," December 1, 2010, http://www.gavialliance.org/library/news/roi/2010/china-s-dramatic-fall-in-hepatitis-b-infections/.

distributes grants and concessional loans—with zero or low interest paid over 25–40 years—to the 81 poorest countries, 39 of which are in Africa.[56] These funds provide support for health, part of a broader category of funding for health, nutrition, and population (HNP). For fiscal years 2009–2012, IDA committed $4.2 billion to health, about 7 percent of its total resources. IBRD lending for health during the period amounted to $8.3 billion, roughly 6.7 percent of IBRD resources.[57]

Nearly 65 percent of IDA funding comes from the governments of its 172 member countries. Every three years, donors meet to replenish IDA resources and review its policy framework. The 16th and most recent replenishment, finalized in 2010, resulted in pledges totaling $49.3 billion dedicated to projects approved during the three-year period ending June 30, 2014. The United States is the largest and most influential World Bank shareholder; its $4.1 billion pledge to IDA 16 accounted for 16 percent of the total. Negotiations on the 17th replenishment will unfold and be concluded over the course of 2013.

The International Finance Corporation (IFC) has expanded its investments in health since 2007. IFC committed almost $2 billion to health projects in 2007-2012, up from $474 million in 2001-2006. In sub-Saharan Africa, IFC commitments grew from $12 million in 2001-2006 to $300 million in 2007-2012.[58] The increase followed an analysis that showed that approximately 50% of health services in the region were provided by the private sector.

Unlike most other development multilateral institutions, the World Bank Group reaches across a broad spectrum of both low- and middle-income countries. Its multisectoral approach to development and poverty alleviation encompasses finance, health, education, transport, and agriculture, among others, which gives the Bank a unique bully pulpit and a special capacity to integrate planning. With its wide-ranging access to heads of state, finance ministers, and other cabinet officers, along with the private sector and increasingly civil-society groups, it can shape countries' choices, encouraging low- and middle-income countries to give health a visibly higher priority, and to make significant, long-term commitments to creating effective health systems. It is able to draw on its expertise in health financing, pensions, taxation, public/private insurance schemes, supply chains, and data management to track investments against the delivery of health services and actual health impacts.

The Bank can point to considerable expertise gained through partnerships in such countries as Mexico, Thailand, Brazil, Turkey, and more recently Rwanda and Burundi, which focused on sustainable health financing, effective and affordable delivery of core health services, and building the systems for ensuring accountability and impacts.

---

56. World Bank, "International Development Association: The World Bank's Fund for the Poorest," http://www.worldbank.org/ida/what-is-ida/fund-for-the-poorest.pdf.

57. Author communication with Melanie Mayhew, Communications Officer, World Bank, January 24, 2013.

58. Author communication with Melanie Mayhew, Communications Officer, World Bank, February 2, 2013.

Policy Developments under the First Obama Administration

As the first Obama term unfolded, the Bank was in the early stages of implementing its 10-year health program, "Healthy Development: The World Bank Strategy for Health, Nutrition and Population Results," launched in 2007.[59] The strategy focuses on preventing poverty as a result of illness and supporting country efforts to develop well-organized, sustainable health systems. It acknowledges the change in the global health architecture in the first decade of the 2000s, noting the proliferation of multilateral organizations, initiatives, and foundations that began financing health programs during the period.

Much of the funding from outside the Bank, it notes, prioritizes specific diseases such as malaria, tuberculosis, and HIV/AIDS, with less focus on broader categories such as health systems and maternal and child health. The Bank stakes out a comparative advantage in strengthening health systems along with health financing and economics and supporting government leadership. While emphasizing system strengthening, the strategy also notes the need for measured outcomes.

Bank commitments over 2009–2012 reflect the strategy's emphasis on systems, with nearly 60 percent of lending devoted to health through the IDA and IBRD focused on "health system performance" (see chart). In line with the three health-specific Millennium Development Goals (MDGs), the Bank has prioritized access to providing reproductive health services; scaling up support for early childhood nutrition; and preventing HIV/AIDS and other communicable diseases.[60]

World Bank Funding Commitments for Health, Nutrition and Population (FY09-FY12)

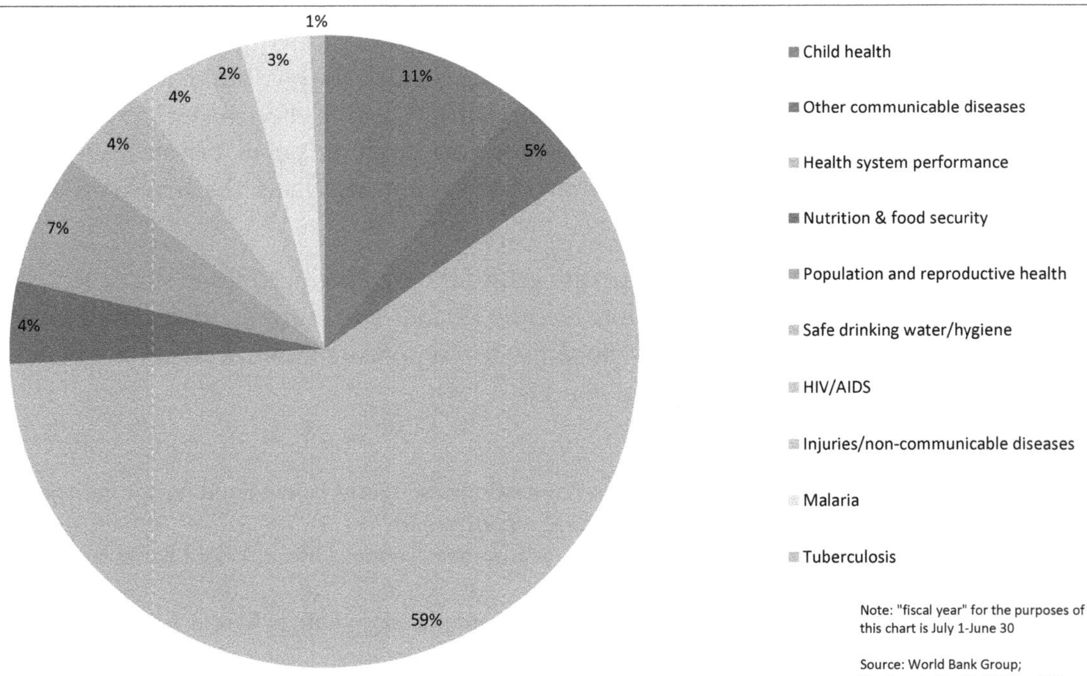

Note: "fiscal year" for the purposes of this chart is July 1-June 30

Source: World Bank Group; Chart created by Matt Fisher, CSIS

59. World Bank, "Healthy Development: the World Bank Strategy for Health, Nutrition, and Population Results," April 24, 2007, http://siteresources.worldbank.org/HEALTHNUTRITIONANDPOPULATION/Resources/281627-1154048816360/HNPStrategyFINALApril302007.pdf.

60. Author communication with Melanie Mayhew, Communications Officer, World Bank, January 11, 2013.

www.ingramcontent.com/pod-product-compliance
Ingram Content Group UK Ltd.
Pitfield, Milton Keynes, MK11 3LW, UK
UKHW051418150926
475561UK00005B/236